7 Days to *Style*

A Guide To Your Authentic Style

By
Monica Diaz
Style Matters, Inc.

Copyright © 2010 by Monica Diaz

All rights reserved. No part of this book may be reproduced, stored, or transmitted by any means—whether auditory, graphic, mechanical, or electronic—without written permission of both publisher and author, except in the case of brief excerpts used in critical articles and reviews. Unauthorized reproduction of any part of this work is illegal and is punishable by law.

ISBN - 13: 978-0-578-05625-8

7 Days to *Style*

This book is dedicated to all the stylish women in my life and a couple of very stylish men. To my mom whose love I can always count on. My sister who I know will always have my back. My dad who was my biggest fan. My friend Ray whose talent and style I admire. All of my friends and family whose love and support mean the world to me and actually make me feel stylish. And finally my style icon, my niece Karina, who knows that a tiara and shiny shoes go with everything.

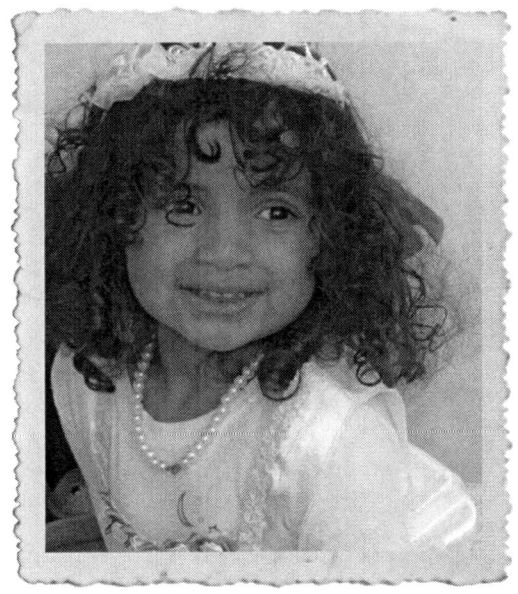

xoxo,
Monica

Contents

Acquiring Style 1

Why Be Stylish? 9

Day 1: Discovering You 17

Day 2: How Others See You 29

Day 3: Shaping Your Style 37

Day 4: Stylish Color 53

Day 5: Stylish Closets 67

Day 6: Let's Make-Up 77

Day 7: Shop Till You Drop 91

Acquiring Style:
Because there's a lot more to style than clothes.

Allow me to introduce myself. My name is Monica Diaz and I was the girl that was overweight, had thick glasses, a bad haircut and an overbite.

Yep, I was a real live *Ugly Betty*. I even wore an authentic Ecuadorian poncho to NYC public school. I had the same bright eyed and bushy tailed attitude that *Betty* has as well. I was teased at school and had no idea why. In my head I was cute and friendly. Why would anyone want to beat me up?!?

Thank goodness, my sister was always there to rescue me. Older, thinner and shy, she too wore a poncho, but no one wanted to kill her. Go figure. Little did the other kids know that they probably could have killed us both – neither of us knew how to fight. The funny part is, we never really got into a fight, and still today, my sister will comment, "I don't know why everyone wanted to beat you up. You were so cute!"

We had and still have a special confidence that I thank God for everyday. We were raised to believe that since we were in the USA we could be whatever we wanted to be. There was nothing stopping us, except ourselves. We just needed to work hard and never feel intimidated by those who were ignorant or intolerant of our diversity.

When I turned 12, things changed overnight. All of a sudden I was chesty, really chunky and just plain unattractive. I was in shock! To make matters worse, my fellow classmates let me know just how unattractive I was everyday. They commented on my weight, my breasts and everything in between. I in turn shrugged them off and kept reading Jane Austin and every other romantic novel imaginable, because I knew in my heart that I was beautiful! Yes, I was hurt and felt ugly at times, but in my heart I was gorgeous. And a little Polly Anna-ish, too.

I wore lots of pink and lace and hair bows. My hair was unruly, my glasses red and I looked like most normal teenage girls–a mess! I wanted to fit in and be just like all my friends, but instead of looking better, I started looking worse! Still, I had a pep in my step and glimmer in my eye. I knew I was cool. I started reading *Seventeen* magazine and then *Vogue* and I fell in love... with fashion.

My love affair grew with every September issue, and then I started to want to look like a model. I could not identify with any of them except Phoebe Cates. She was the closest to an Ecuadorian-looking model I could find, and I loved her.

I had not realized that something in me was changing. For the first time, I had wanted to look like someone else, someone other than me. It is at this point in our lives as girls when we often start losing confidence in ourselves, trying to look like a model, a movie star, a popular girl in school. It is at this point in our lives as young women that we start getting image complexes. I was no exception.

All my friends were thin and could wear anything they wanted. I, of course, thought I could as well. So, I decided I was going to buy all the clothes I could afford with my part-time work money. My plan: buy super cheap and buy a lot. Well, not that much, since I did not have that much money to begin with.

Both my parents started to get tired of my cheap, ill-fitting outfits. My mother, who is not one to keep her thoughts to herself, let me have it at age 15. You see, the 15th birthday for a Latina is extremely important. This is the day she becomes a young lady, no longer a child.

It literally was that drastic. Before then, it used to be that you were not allowed to wear anything that was close to be being "teenage stylish". No heels, no make-up, no nail polish, no nothing.

One evening my mom sat me down and gave it to me straight. It went something like this: "You have to stop buying all these cheap clothes that make you look cheap and get ruined after the first wash. You need to start wearing quality clothes that make you look and feel attractive and classy. We are going shopping tomorrow". There was a lot more said, believe me, but I prefer the paraphrased short version.

Mind you, my mother worked in a factory. She wore heels and a dress to work and then changed when she got to the factory. So to her it was unacceptable that I, a young lady going to school and working part-time, could not look "put together".

So, off we went to a boutique in our neighborhood. This place was chic and the really pretty girls shopped there. I was excited! I can remember it like it was yesterday. I tried on a pair of pale sea-foam green light wool trousers, an emerald green thin silk shirt and burgundy high heel shoes. I came out, looked at myself in the mirror, and thought, "Wow, I love this." I can still see my mom sitting in the boutique with a huge smile that said, "This is how you should look all the time. This is you". She bought me the complete outfit! She said, "It is not how many clothes you have. It is the quality that is important".

That outfit changed my image. I loved the way I felt and looked in my new clothes. I felt sophisticated and in charge. I felt like me. I started dieting and exercising and morphing into a young lady.

The fact that I saw myself in something that well put together made me realize I had goals and I needed the clothes to get me there. I was not trying to copy anyone else. *I was being me.*

Now, don't get me wrong. I had plenty of fashion mistakes after that, or like my dad used like to say, "*Mi hija,* remember when you used to dress really bad?" I refused to admit I was ever anything but stylish, although I must agree now that not all my vintage clothing choices were good ones.

So you see, you are not necessarily born with style, but you can acquire it. It is the love that you have for yourself that propels you to better yourself internally and externally. For me, these and many other experiences molded not only my personality but also my style. The more I grew as a person, the more style I acquired.

Style comes from self-discovery. It comes from a confidence and love of yourself. Style is an expression of who you are that is silent and extremely loud at the same time. You are not saying a word, but your clothes and image are screaming a message that is very loud and clear.

I started writing about my childhood so that you can better understand me. I can tell you all of my career credentials, but knowing who I am and where I come from gives you a better idea of why I really wrote this book. Like that time in the boutique when I first saw the way I looked in the mirror matching the way I thought about myself, I love the look I see in my clients, whether it is a seminar or a private consultation. They make that same magical discovery about themselves. It is the look of knowing you are worth it, you can look fantastic, and yes, you can express your true self through your appearance. But this happens only when the person truly trusts the process that we go through together.

I love my business because I get to share my love and knowledge of fashion while helping others gain confidence, save time and save money. They will no longer stand in front of a messy closet thinking, "I have nothing to wear", or go shopping just because there is a sale, spending a ridiculous amount of money on unnecessary things. Or worse, look at themselves and dislike what they see.

This book is an abridged version of the process I go through with my private clients. I work with them first to discover who they are and then we start building and creating an image that reflects their true selves and their goals. I am sure you have read plenty of fashion and style books before, but what makes *7 Days To Style* different is that you get to do something everyday to discover who you truly are and reveal the true you. *In 7 days you will acquire style, YOUR authentic style.*

Before you start the program, I want you to read the book in its entirety. You need to prepare yourself mentally to go through the whole process, plan dates and make appointments in order to make this happen. There are a few pages you might want to make copies of and some that you will need to carry with you.

Remember to be true to yourself and be open to change.

"No man should part with his own individuality and become that of another."

– William Ellery Channing

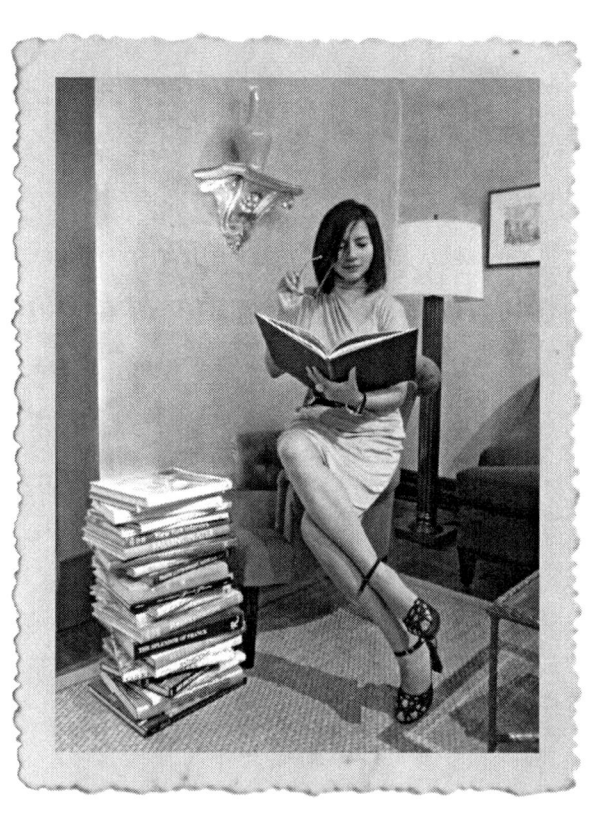

Why Be Stylish?

"When the student is ready, the teacher will appear."

– Chinese proverb

This Chinese proverb is one of my favorites. I truly believe that when you are ready to learn something new and make a positive change, all of the pieces start to fall into place. The stars align and the right people and situations appear serendipitously. When I first thought about starting a business, I had a lot of different ideas. The one thing I knew, though, was that I needed to do something I loved and something that would benefit others. I knew that I loved fashion and teaching.

I was always asked by friends and family to help with fashion choices. They admired my style, and because I am a fashion professional, they respected my opinion. After working the process with them, I saw my friends beginning to see their true selves for the first time. I saw them beginning to gain confidence as they saw how amazing they looked. They were ready to conquer the world! So, that was the start of my business, Style Matters, Inc.

True style is not just about clothing. There is a lot more to style than clothes. *True style is about embracing who you are, as you are, and enhancing your attributes in order to exude your natural elegance.*

This book caught your attention because you are ready for a change. You are ready to start investing in yourself and shine. I am sure you have seen a makeover show and secretly thought, "I want to be that woman". Well, this is *your time* to be her. The only thing stopping you is *you*. You are ready to start and I am ready to teach you!

Get ready to start on a fun journey that will take you from average to stylish. In order for you to get the most out of this workbook, you need to keep an open mind. I meet with clients all the time and my best results are always from the ones that trust me and trust the process. It is not always easy, but I assure you it is always fun. The results are incredible and relationships I build always turn into friendships.

The purpose of this book is to guide you through a week of self-discovery and transformation.

Why do you need style?

Your appearance speaks volumes about who you are, even before you say a word. That's right. We all do it. We all judge books by the cover. We classify someone as soon as we see them. We give them an age, education level, social status and marital status. Right or wrong, it is human nature. There have been many studies done on how an individual's first impression can be the deciding factor on whether they get a job or not. Just take a quick look around you next time and see how you seem to gravitate towards certain individuals and tend to not want to associate with others. You have not spoken to any of them, and yet there is that subconscious reaction of making judgments. It is a normal reaction and it is the reason why first impressions are often lasting impressions.

That is why you have to make the best of your appearance. That is why you have to dress for who you aspire to be.

If we know our appearance is important, *why do we neglect it so much?* The answer is a little complicated and there are quite a few factors that come into play. First, there is the fear of change. We are comfortable with our look. What if we change and then hate it? There is also the fear of being exposed. Yes, people hide behind bad fashion choices. They fear not being accepted for who they really are and so they put up a front, a costume of sorts.

Then there are the multiple excuses of money, weight, and time. We think we need to be in perfect shape, have tons of money, and go shopping everyday in order to look great. We hide inside our fear and insecurities and become immobile. We get stuck in a rut. How do we change this?

We get educated!

We learn that in the matters of fashion, money does not matter. Age does not matter. It is *Style* that truly *Matters*. That is where this book comes in.

As personal stylist, I teach individuals how to discover their own unique style and how to express who they are and their goals to others through clothing.

This workbook is based on the step-by-step process that I take my personal clients through. I made this a 7 day process because it will take you some time to put all the pieces together and actually process what you are discovering. You can take a little longer if you like but don't take too long because in my experience, the longer you procrastinate, the more likely you are to quit. You see, change is hard. There is comfort in the known and discomfort in the unknown. You are already stuck and you know you need to move forward, so make yourself and me a promise to start this book and finish it.

And just as I do with my private clients, here is a small contract that I need for you to sign. Keep looking at whenever you start having doubts:

Style Contract

On this date, _____, I make a commitment to myself to take care of myself and be open minded through this process. I promise to do all the exercises in this book. I promise to always think of myself as beautiful and sexy, even when I am having a down day. I will wake up every morning, look in the mirror and see the beautiful woman I have always wanted to be: stylish, strong and gorgeous.

_____
Signature

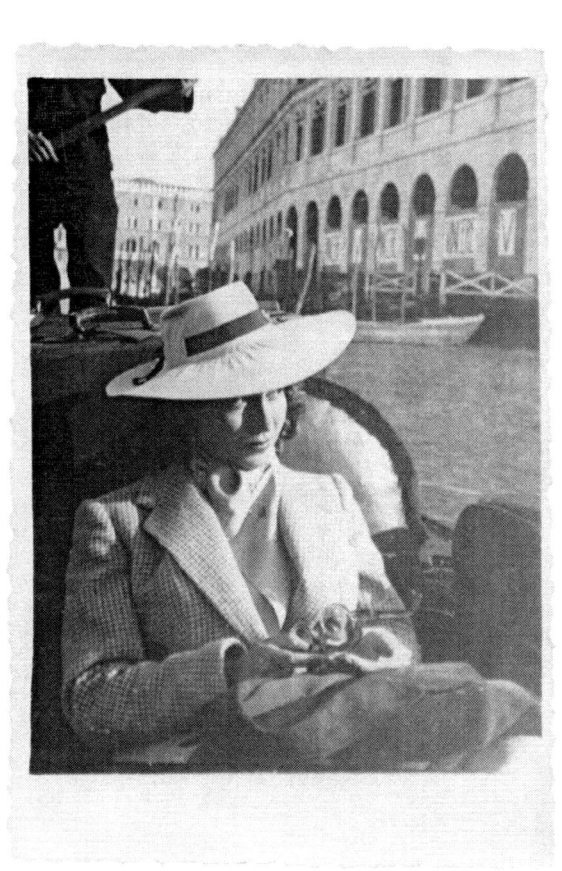

Day 1

"Fashion is general. Style is individual."

– Edan Woolman Chase

Discovering You

Through out this book, I have included quotes that best express the messages I would like you to absorb. One of my favorites is Mary Mcfadden's "Know yourself, then create yourself". This to me describes style. Style is knowing who you are and getting that message across to others.

In today's fashion world, we are so busy trying to get "the look for less" that we ignore whether that look works for us. We are so celebrity-driven that if so-and-so is wearing something, we want to copy it. Remember the Madonna imitators of the late '80s, or the recent celebutante-wanna-be's of the past ten years?

It is one thing if you are a kid. You are supposed to have fun with different looks. That is the time to make mistakes. But for those of us who have already been-there-and-done-that, it is time to move on from the hottest new trend of the last five minutes.

Trends are fashion looks of the moment, while style is eternal.

Personal style is *your* essence. You don't need to look to other people for style. You have your own style, your own signature to make. ***Instead, you need to look to yourself.*** Look inside yourself to discover your own true style.

Have you ever looked at reality show makeovers? There are always a few contestants whose sense of fashion is absurd. You know what I mean. Sometime during the show, those contestants will have a breakdown. What they are having is a breakthrough, a point when they realize that they have been hiding behind clothes or an image that is really not true to them.

That moment is a huge hurdle. People can finally get in touch with their real feelings. They can begin to discover the truth from within. They can begin to learn that true style comes from within. Finally, they can relax, trust, and begin to enjoy the process.

The journey of self-discovery is often an emotional one, but one well worth taking.

This is your journey of self-discovery. I am not going to say that it replaces real therapy but fashion therapy is something I do all the time, and it works. So get ready to be honest and brace yourself for a change.

Discovering Your Style Need

The following questions will help you get a clearer view of your personal style. These questions relate to your lifestyle: What do you truly enjoy? What does your life consist of? Knowing these things will assist you in creating a look that is uniquely you.

Are you happy with your lifestyle?

What do you enjoy doing the most?

What do you hate doing?

What would your ideal lifestyle look like?

Does your wardrobe reflect the life that you have, the life that you want to have, or neither?

How would you describe your style?

Do you travel for business, pleasure, both or neither?

How often to you dine out with family/friends?

Are you a member of a gym or sports club?

Do you have any hobbies, such as cooking or dancing?

Are there some hobbies that you want to develop, such as photography?

Do you belong to any professional organizations or volunteer your time?

What percentage of your time would you say requires business attire?

What percentage of your time requires casual attire?

How often do you go shopping for yourself? Do you enjoy it?

If you could change one thing about your style, what would it be?

What do love about your inner self? Your outer self?
Ex: friendly personality and fantastic legs.

If you could change just one thing about yourself, what would it be?

Your Style Vision Board

This part of the day is the most fun. You get to sit down and create a Style Vision Board of everything you like and aspire to be. A vision board is simply a collage of pictures and images that you love. When you make a vision board dedicated to style, you are letting yourself claim your own sense of style —all the things that make you feel like you. Seeing my clients put together their Style Vision Board is one of my favorite exercises.

Here is what you will need:

Scissors, several fashion magazines (and even home décor and travel magazines, if you have them), a pen, a large piece of paper or poster board, digital camera, printer and glue stick.

- Collect lots of fashion magazines and catalogues. Remember this is about style, so if you have home and travel magazines, you can use them, too. Style is not only what you wear, but how you live and everything that surrounds you.
- Sit down and cut out everything you like. Perhaps the color is fantastic or the actual garment is gorgeous. You might like the feeling a certain picture gives you. Whatever it is, cut it out.
- Remember there are no limitations except the ones you set for yourself. Don't think, "This is couture Chanel and I'll never own it", or "This model is size 0 and I'm not even close". The Style Vision Board is simply about what you love and what you are attracted to. It is not about what you can afford or whether you can wear it. Lead with your heart–not with your head.
- Weed out your collection of pictures down to the 10 you absolutely love. Make sure that at least 6 deal strictly with fashion (as opposed to travel, for instance).

- Tape each photo or image to a large piece of paper, leaving enough space nearby to write a sentence or two.
- Write why you love that particular picture or image in the space nearby.

Look at your Style Vision Board. And now, look at the answers you gave in Discovering Your Style Needs. Do they seem to mesh? How are they different and how are they alike?

If the answers you have seem different than those on your board, then: ***FOLLOW YOUR STYLE VISION BOARD.***

Why? Because your Style Vision Board is your idea of style without limitations. Because sometimes when we answer questions, we may be a bit inhibited, thinking about what the answer should be. Because your Style Vision Board comes from you organically. It is 100% you. It is yours.

Claim it! Write ten words that best describe your style vision that is reflected in your Style Vision Board. Come up with your own words to best describe your style: chic, playful, classic, trendy, young, down to earth, etc.

Once you have written these words, put together a sentence using them.

For example:
"My style is eclectic, free-spirited, yet classic..." because your Style Vision Board reflects your love for all things indigenous, traditional tailoring and travel.

Use My Style Statement worksheet provided on page 24 for your answers.

Style Vision Board

My Style Statement

My Style Vision Boards reflects the following lifestyle, personality and fashion style.

These are the ten best words that describe me and my style.

This is my style statement:

Take a digital photo of your Vision Board. Print it out. Paste it in to the space provided on the next page. Whenever you like, you can look at it to remind you of your own style vision and aspirations.

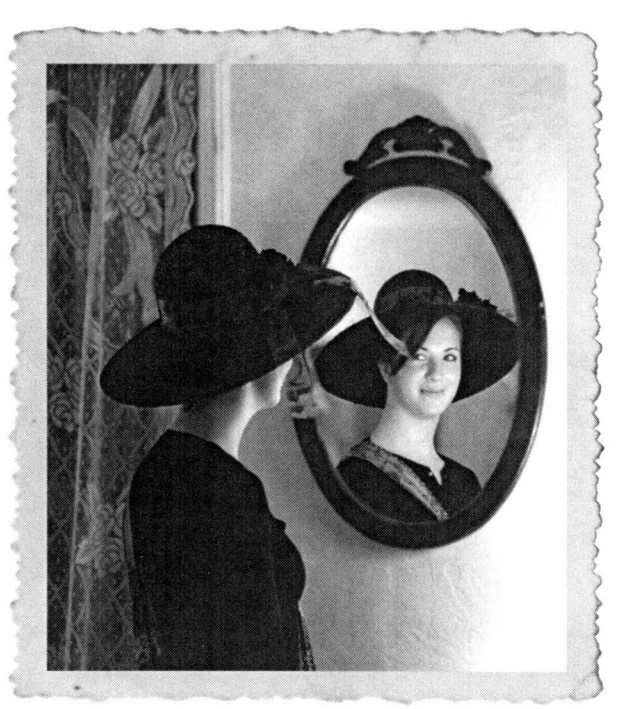

Day 2

"Style is a reflection of your attitude and your personality."

– Shawn Ashmore

How others see me

You now have an idea of what your appearance expresses to others, but you might still be a bit confused. Getting an outsider's point of view is always important.

At this point in your *7 Days to Style,* I want you to ask some people whose opinion you trust to answer a few questions about you. The questions are very general and open-ended so that the person has an opportunity to elaborate. Consider asking people whose fashion style you like but who will also be honest. This might be hard, but be open to their critique, listen to their answers and most importantly, do not speak or get defensive. Just be open and grateful to get feedback. Use the worksheet later on in this chapter to record their answers.

Questions:

How would you describe my style?
What is my best feature?
Which of my current outfits looks best on me?
What color do I wear that looks great on me?
Do you think my personality matches my fashion style?
Do you think my hair and make up look good on me?
What do you think others say when they first meet me?
Do you think I dress younger or older than my age?
Does my fashion match my career?
If you could change one thing about my fashion style, what would it be?

These questions will give you a very clear view of how others see you.

Ideally, you should ask at least three people, but if this makes you too uncomfortable, please be sure to ask one. This is so important because these exercises allow you to get an idea of what others see. I do believe that everyone has at least one good friend who will be honest and kind. I actually prefer that you ask someone whom you are not too close with, because that person will often be more honest. A coworker, for instance, is someone that sees you everyday, and chances are, you have a friendly-enough relationship to ask these questions, but you two are probably not so close emotionally that you would take the feedback personally. The feedback is probably less likely to feel hurtful.

You might want to start the conversation by saying something like:

"Hey _____, I am trying to tweak my image a little and I want to get your honest opinion on a few things. I trust your opinion and like your style so I would love your feedback. Do you have a few minutes?"

Day 2 is a little difficult I know, but it really is helpful. Understanding how we see ourselves and how others see us is extremely important when it comes to finding your own style.

You must remember that personal style is not about pleasing others or about wearing the trendiest clothes. **Personal style is about being true to yourself,** confident and able to dress in a manner that both best expresses your personality and enhances your best features.

What They Said

_____ said:

What I Feel and Think of the Comments:

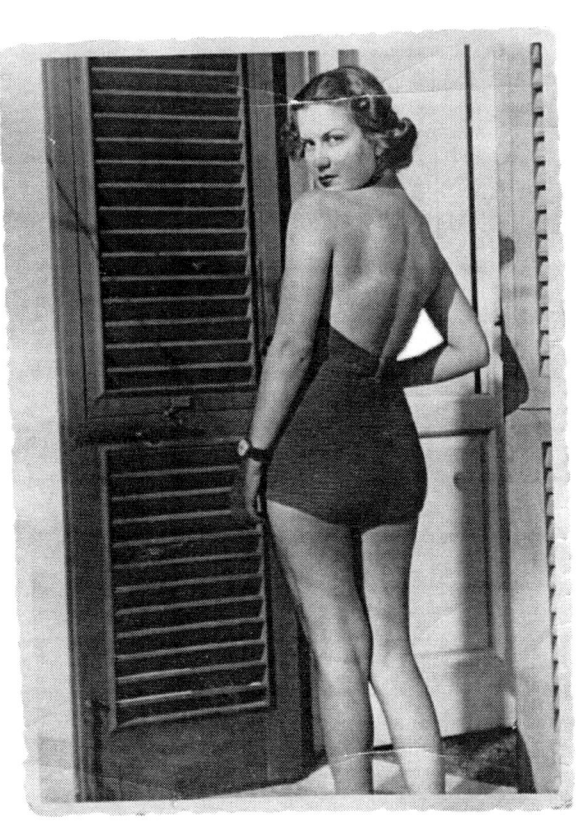

Day 3

"Curve: The loveliest distance between two points."

– Mae West

Shaping Your Style

Understanding a woman's silhouette is the key to knowing how to dress. Your silhouette is the outline of your body. Many have compared women's bodies to different fruit or geometric shapes. I find that almost depressing. Hearing someone say "I'm pear shaped" or "I'm built like a ruler", how B-O-R-I-N-G! Please! We are speaking about *our bodies*, the ones we use everyday to express our emotions, carry our children and seduce our lovers. See what I mean? How can we compare it to a triangle?

As you already know, I'm Latina. This means many things to many people and lots of foregone conclusions. The one truth is yes, we are passionate individuals, yes we are expressive and yes we do love curves on women. So with that said, I am going to take a Latin approach and compare women's silhouettes to musical instruments. You see, when a woman is all gorgeous and curvy in Latin America is she compared to a guitar. How romantic, *(sigh)*.

I always wanted to be that guitar but I had another musical sound inside of me. I like to think that we each have our own music to make, our own rhythm that we need to dance. Have you ever walked down the street with your Ipod on? Your favorite song is playing and all of a sudden you are walking quicker or slower depending on the beat and swaying a little because you want to dance. You forget about your body issues and you just want to move. You should feel that way everyday when you put on a great outfit because it is allowing you to play that music.

To find out your silhouette's music, you do not need to take your measurements. You just need to stand in front of the mirror in your lingerie, look at yourself endearingly and listen to the music your body is playing. Will you hear the sounds of a Guitar, Harp, Mandolin or Saxophone?

To get started, answer the questions on the Style Profile worksheet and then take a look at the Musical Style in order to understand your silhouette.

Note: I know that many of you think that if you gain weight, you will fall into a different category, but the truth is that your shape stays the same. You will still be the same shape if you are a size six or a sixteen. So don't worry. **Your true melody never changes.**

Style Profile

My Basic Information

The following information is designed to help you identify your shape, so please answer them honestly. There will be no tape measure involved, just an honest visual analysis. Try not to be too hard on yourself. Stand in front of a full-length mirror in your lingerie.

Height:

Weight:

Current Dress size:

Circle the best letter below:

Shoulders	a) Wider than hips	b) Balanced with hips	c) Narrower than hips
Bust	a) Full	b) Small	c) Average
Waist	a) Smaller than bust	b) About same as bust	c) Larger than bust
Hips	a) Narrow	b) Larger than bust & waist	c) About same as bust

Below are some of the combinations that correspond to each body type.

Guitar: B+B+A+C or B+C+A+C
Harp: A+A+C+A
Mandolin: C+C+B+B or C+B+B+B
Saxophone: B+B+B+C

Now think about your figure. List:

What I LOVE about my figure:

What I should try to downplay:

What should I try to enhance:

Musical Style

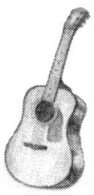

Guitar: *Gorgeous and Graceful:* This woman has curves! Rounded hips, full bust and well defined waist. Her weight gain is evenly distributed.

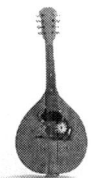

Harp: *Harmonious and Heavenly:* This woman has beautiful ample shoulders and slim shapely legs. Her waist is not that well defined and she carries her weight in her upper body.

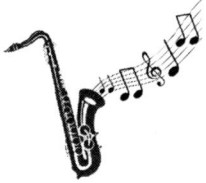

Mandolin: *Melodious and Modern:* This woman has a beautiful small waist, full rounded hips, and a relatively flat stomach. Her shoulders are narrow in comparison to her hips. She gains weight first her lower body and very rarely her upper body.

Saxophone: *Slight and Sultry:* This woman has a slender body with small breasts, narrow hips and an undefined waist. Like the guitar, she gains weight evenly. This woman, with her lack of curves, is often called the ideal fashion plate.

Stylish Dressing

Now that you have learned the music your body plays, here is a small list of do's and don'ts.

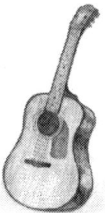

Guitar

You have beautiful curves that need to be shown. Your proportions are balanced and you have to do very little to be bombshell gorgeous. Your objective is to keep your look balanced. Do not hide your curves under baggy clothes. Baggy clothes will just add extra pounds to your figure. You will want to pick fabrics that hug your curves, not tightly, but just barely skimming the body. Your fashion silhouettes should imitate your shape and be curvy. Nothing straight for you. Monochromatic color looks will make you appear taller and slimmer.

Jackets & Coats:
Tailored fitted jackets nipped at the waist are very flattering on you. Try single breasted jackets with either two or three buttons. Belted jackets that fall below the hip are great for Guitars that want to minimize their bottoms. A single breasted, nicely tailored coat is beautiful on your shape.

Pants:
Traditional flat front trousers are a fine look for you since they accentuate your waist and hips. A flair leg works great as well to balance your curves. Jeans with traditional boot leg or a flair leg are also flattering on you. If you feel comfortable in shorts, wear them either short or Bermuda-style.

Skirts:
Follow the same rules as trousers. Keep the waist band a little low and the fit skimming the body. Pencil skirts look fabulous as do trouser style, A-line, circle and bias cut skirts. Mini skirts work for you, but be careful. Because you have curves, these skirts may look too short. I especially like sarong or wrap skirts for you, too, as they will skim your curves.

Tops:
Again, think softly curved skimming styles. Choose simple styles that will not add too much bulk on top. Silk blouses that drape softly will look fabulous on you. Wrap tops are a natural for you in a deep "V" with soft textures. Halters look great on you especially with "V" neck lines to open up the front line. Turtle necks work nicely if you have a long or average neck. Make sure to use mock turtle necks if you have a short neck. T-shirts should not be too tight or too short because they create an unsophisticated look. A better T-shirt style is a hip length body skimming shape.

Dresses:
Look for body-conscious simple lines. Silhouettes that show off your waist and legs work beautifully. A V-neck elongates the torso and belts emphasize your small waist. My favorite classic look for all shapes is a sheath dress. Yours should be shapely and nipped at the waist with a belt. Wrap dresses are my favorite, because they are just so sexy and you can make them work. Biased cut dresses shape the body beautifully. Strapless is also a nice look, but if you have a full bust make sure to wear a great bra, fitted by a professional.

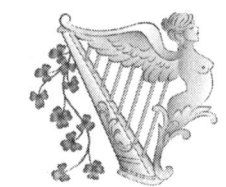

Harp

You have strong shoulders, an ample bust and beautiful legs that need to be shown off. You do not need any shoulder pads or anything that adds bulk to your already beautifully strong shoulders. In order not to appear too top heavy, you need to keep tops simple. You can, however, play with detailing on your pants or skirts. Lucky for you–you can wear mini skirts and skinny jeans.

Jackets & Coats:
Tailored jackets should have a soft line shoulder pads. Keep the lapels small. Peak lapels will just accentuate your shoulders too much. Mandarin collar skirt jackets look very nice on you. Make sure the fit is not tight, as that will accentuate your bust-line. An ideal jacket length for you is at the hipbone. For coats, try below the knee. A nice classic A-line coast works well, as do pea coats and sweater/cardigan coats.

Pants:
You are lucky that you can wear almost any pant style. Since you have narrow hips, pants that hit your hips look very flattering. Narrow skinny pants look great, as do wide leg trousers. With jeans, you can play with pocket detailing to draw attention and add curves to your bottom. Shorts will look fabulous on you. Just make sure that when you wear shorts or minis, your tops are not too snug or revealing.

Skirts:
I love pencil skirts and A-line skirts on all shapes but yours can especially carry them off. Wrap skirts and pleated skirts work well, because they add curves to your bottom.

Tops:
Here is where you have to be careful because you do not want to add too much volume to this area. Soft silhouettes with soft shoulders work best. Keep details to a minimum and make sure that the sleeves are not puffy or have horizontal lines. Tailored shirts look elegant on you. V- and U-cut tops will elongate your neckline and slim you. Wrap tops will work if you get styles that are longer and not too bulky around the middle. The idea is to create length. T-shirt and turtle necks look good when they skim the body, and are not too tight.

Dresses:
Follow the rules of body-conscious simple lines. Silhouettes that show off your legs work beautifully. Semi-fitted shift dresses and tunic dresses look fabulous on you. Styles that are belted at the hip work well because they emphasis your narrowest area: your hips. A strapless dress looks great since it focuses on your sexy shoulders. Wrap dresses help you create the illusion of curves and coat dresses give you an easy professional look. Add a belt to a dress in order to give the illusion of a tinier waist.

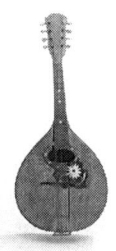

Mandolin

Your body has all the soft curves at the bottom. Your torso is slim and your bust is small. Your aim is to create the illusion of a more balanced silhouette by adding volume to your top while keeping your lower half simple. If your shoulders are narrow or sloped, add shoulder pads to create more volume. You have beautiful rounded hips and may or may not have a rounded derriere, which means you want to keep your silhouette soft and body-slimming.

Jackets & Coats:
Tailored jackets should have a soft line and shoulder pads. You can do peaked lapels which accentuate and widen your shoulders. Belted cardigan-style jackets work well on you, as do bomber and short jackets that emphasis the upper body. Chanel-style jackets that are cropped look wonderful and very elegant. Your coats should have an A-line to skim your bottom half and shape your upper body. Military and trench coats work well when belted, since they emphasize your tiny waist.

Pants:
Since you have a shapely lower body, you do not need to do much. Trousers with a straight or wide leg work best. Keep it simple — no embellishments or too much stitching details as this draws attention to your bottom. Side pockets add bulk to your hips, as do back pockets. If you love the look of a side pocket trouser, you can opt for keeping the pocket sewn shut. You can actually do a flare or wide leg pant if the line comes

straight and smooth down the front. Be careful not to do a skinny jean or legging since this will really look unflattering. You also need to be careful with cropped and short pants because they can cut off your silhouette and add bulk to your bottom.

Skirts:
Keep the style simple. I like A-line skirts best for you because they grace your shape nicely and look fabulous. A pencil skirt could be tricky if it is loose at the waist. The solution is to have it tailored to fit you properly. (Many women are unaware or afraid of getting their clothing tailored, but it really is key for a perfect fit.) Ask your dry cleaner for a referral. Make sure that skirts do not have any buckles or ties at the hip, which will add bulk.

Tops:
This is where you can play and add embellishments. I like full sleeves and shoulder treatments for a Mandolin body. Horizontal boat neck sailor tops are fabulous on you. Ballet neck and square necks are also good looks for you because they create a horizontal line that adds volume, which balances your lower body. You are lucky; you can do bulky turtlenecks while others have to stay away. You can wear cable knits and fisherman knits nicely.

Dresses:
You look great in empire wait dresses since they follow your natural shape. I would add a nice padded bra to lift and draw attention to your décolletage. Wrap dresses and slight A-line dresses work for you as well since they follow your curves. A straight sheath dress works when it has a fuller shaped bottom. A dress cut too straight will be ill-fitting, since it goes against your natural body contours.

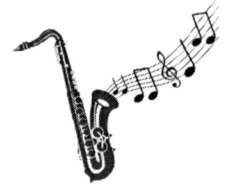

Saxophone

You may not have lots of curves, but your body was made for sashaying down the catwalk. You can wear almost anything, but you need to be careful not to choose clothes that make you look too boyish. You have a slim frame and you will want to create the illusion of curves. You can wear mini skirts and skinny jeans, but you need to wear them with tops that are girly and fun, or tailored and sexy.

Jackets & Coats:
Look for tailored styles that have a nipped waist to create the illusion of a well-defined waistline. Belted jackets have the same effect, since they nip the jacket to emphasis the waist. If you have a thick waist, though, be careful. You will want to look for straighter styles that follow your shape. Mandarin collar shirt jackets look very nice on you. If you are short-waisted, make sure that the jacket's belt hit you a little above your natural waist. A great jacket length for you is at the hipbone. For coats, have them fall below the knee. A nice classic coat works well, as do pea coats and sweater/cardigan coats.

Pants:
You, as well as the Harp girl, are very lucky: you can wear almost any pant style. Since you have narrow hips, pants that hit your hips look very flattering on you. Narrow, skinny pants look fantastic, as do wide leg trousers. You can play with pocket detailing on your jeans. This will draw the attention to your bottom, giving the illusion of curves. Shorts will look stunning, as will minis, since you legs are usually slim.

Skirts:
You can definitely wear a fuller skirt that adds volume to your bottom. A-line and pencil skirts work on all shapes and look slimming and sexy. If your bust is small-to-average, you can usually do a high-waisted style. Wrap skirts and pleated skirts give you a sexy curved silhouette.

Tops:
Top styles depend upon whether you have a small waist. A loose fitting blouse looks best if your waist is thick, since it will drape nicely. If you are slim all over, dare to wear bulky sweaters. They will look awesome on you. On all saxophones, tailored shirts look sophisticated, and wrap tops will create an illusion of feminine curves.

Dresses:
Silhouettes that show off your legs work beautifully. Semi-fitted shift dresses and tunic dresses look fabulous on you. Styles that are belted at the hip or at the waist all look flattering. Strapless dresses, wrap dresses and coat dresses all work—how lucky!

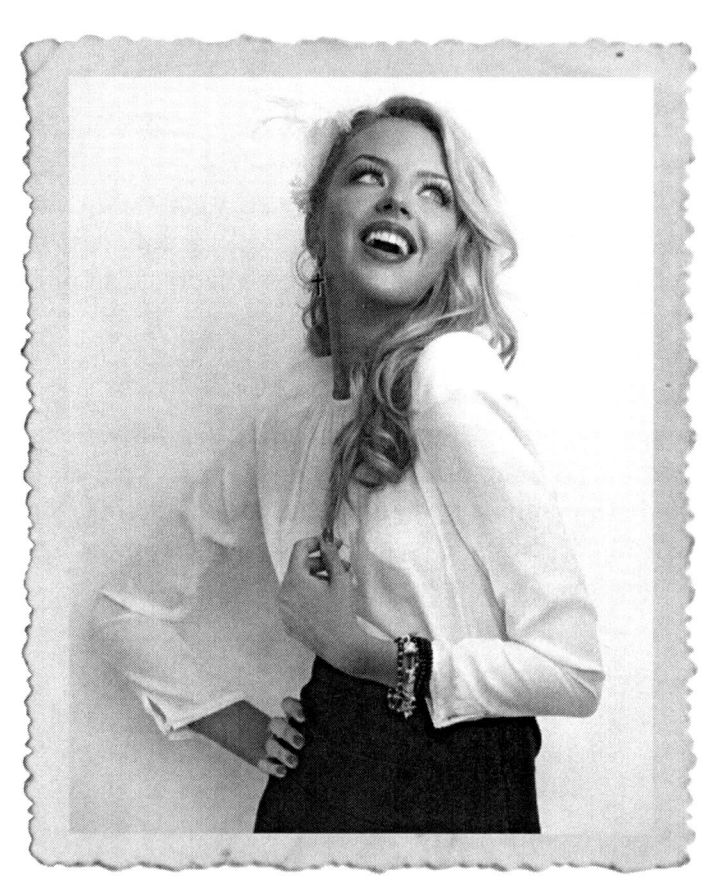

Day 4

"The best color in the whole world is the one that looks good on you!"

– Coco Chanel

Stylish Color

"Which colors do you think look best?" This is one of the questions I hear all the time. There are many color theories and I do believe that they work. Unfortunately, they are very complicated and almost impossible for people to learn overnight. Instead, I will simplify them. This will help you understand color better and the importance of wearing the ones that work best for you.

Let me start by saying that color has the power to make you look radiant or just plan dull. How many times do people comment on how great that color looks on you? Probably not so much, because if they had, you would be wearing it a lot more! Here in NYC, we are almost afraid of color. We stick with our black uniform because it is easy and we think it looks chic. Well, black done right *can* be chic, but like any other trend, it can also look boring.

Why else does color matter? Color has the power to evoke emotion. It can actually make you feel better. So let's put our fear of color aside, and let's start making ourselves feel and look better!

You may have heard of people being categorized as a season – spring, summer, winter, or fall– depending on their hair, skin and eye color. This is perhaps the simplest color analysis theory and one that I will explain in a simplified way in this book.

There are three basic things to keep in mind. Colors can either have cool undertones, which have more blue pigments, or warm undertones, which have more yellow pigments. Then, there is the value or depth of color. This refers to lightness or darkness of a color. The next thing to consider is the intensity of color, or how bright or muted a color is.

Generally, people are basically divided into either cool or warm undertones, and either low or high contrast coloring.

In order for you to know which colors look best, you will need to take three tests that will give you a better understanding of how colors work for you. There are so many colors in the rainbow that it would be impossible for me to give a list of each and every color, but if you have a sense of the basic ideas of what to look for, you will not need a list. Ever.

Also, take into consideration your personality when choosing colors. A bubbly personality will wear stronger colors better than a more reserved personality.

After taking these tests and playing with colors, you will start to see which colors work best for you. The cosmetics or make-up colors you choose will also depend on the results of these tests. You can wear any color you like, but try to keep the colors that flatter you around your face. The face is the most expressive partof the body, and the right color will let it radiate its beauty.

Color Test

First Test: Warm or cool undertone.

You will need to get either two pieces of fabric or two pieces jewelry. Of the two pieces, one must be gold and the other silver. Once you have these, put on a strapless bra or wrap a towel around your top, and sit in front of a well lit mirror.

Start by either draping the gold or silver piece around your neck so that it is close to your face. If you are working with jewelry make sure that it is a thick enough necklace or big enough earrings so that you can get an accurate reading.

Keep alternating between the gold and the silver to determine which one looks best. Take notice of how your skin tone will actually look more radiant with one more than the other.

If the gold looks best, you have warm undertones. If the silver looks best, you have cool undertones.

Second Test: Warm or cool undertone.

Sometimes the gold-or-silver test is not enough. Some may need to see themselves in nonmetallic colors. For this test, you will need two different cloths, one in orange and the other in hot pink. If you do not have garments in these colors, then go to a department store and try on some tops. Again, you are looking to see which color actually adds a glow to your skin, as opposed to making you look sallow.

If orange looks good, you have warm undertones. If hot pink looks good, you have cool undertones.

Third Test: Value/Intensity

This test will decide the value and depth of the color you should wear. It will help you determine if you look better in muted or intense colors.

For those individuals with warm undertones, you will need to use an orange fabric and a peach fabric. For those individuals with cool undertones, use a hot pink fabric and a soft pink fabric.

Again, drape the color around your face and determine which one is more harmonious with your over all coloring.

If you looked better in the stronger color, your coloring is high intensity. If the softer color looked better, your coloring is low intensity.

Wearing Color

Warm & Low Intensity
You have gold undertones with clear and bright coloring. You look better in ivory or eggshell than in pure white. When choosing a red you need to make sure it has a yellow undertone so that it looks a bit orange. You look great in green and yellow. Soft aqua and peach are also flattering. Try to look for clear, not muted, colors. Think of the soft palette of spring pastels. Gold is your metal. This combination is known as Spring.

Warm & High Intensity
You have gold undertones with dark coloring. Your best white is also ivory or eggshell, as pure white will overpower you. Your red should also be yellow-based, leaning more towards an orange. Your best colors are mustard, evergreen, rust and orange. Think of the beautiful colors of the fall foliage. Colors should be muted, and not too bright. Avoid pink. Peach is your color. This combination is known as Autumn.

Cool & Low Intensity
Your undertones are blue, making a true white a better choice than ivory. Your jewelry looks best when it is silver. You have soft and muted coloring. Reds that are blue based look best on you, as do soft powdered and muted colors. Grays, cornflower blue, navy and dusty rose all work on you. This combination is known as Summer.

Cool & High Intensity
Your coloring is clear and dramatic. You have blue undertones and therefore look best in pure white, and silver your best metal. You should look for vivid colors. Think of the deep intense colors of jewel tones and winter. Your reds should be true ruby red. Burgundy, teal, navy, grey and purple all look great on you.

Pink and fuchsia look better on you than peach and orange. This combination is known as Winter.

Color Worksheet

RESULTS OF COLOR TEST

My natural hair color is:

My natural eye color is:

My natural skin tone is:

My undertone is:

My color intensity is:

My wardrobe consists of the following colors:

After knowing which colors look best on me, I feel my color choices are (good/poor and explain):

The following are changes I plan to make when selecting color in my wardrobe:

Musical Style, Meet Style Rules: the marriage of color, lines, and texture

In order to create the desired results which best flatter your silhouette, you need to understand a little about color, lines and texture. Designers use these simple rules to create their collections. In essence, this is the basics of design and it will help you with all your fashion choices.

Color

Colors can create a mood. They make us happy, blue, excited or relaxed and are even used for therapy. In design, colors work to enhance our beauty and add to the illusion of a perfect body.

Light colors reflect light, causing the covered area to appear larger. When worn with dark colors, the eye is attracted to the light area. If you wear a light color around your face, the eye is drawn to the face.

Dark colors absorb light, causing the covered area to appear smaller. This is the reason that dark colors are used to make the figure appear slimmer. Dark colors de-emphasize the size of the body. If you have a sallow skin tone, dark colors make you appear tired.

Bright colors attract attention to the covered area. This is the reason why bright colors are used for certain uniforms. When worn with a dark color, the bright color stands out, and the viewer's eye is attracted to the bright color.

Lines

Vertical lines make the eye travel up and down the frame. This makes the area covered appear slimmer and longer, and about 90% of the time, this is the look we strive for.

Horizontal lines make the eye travel across the covered area. The area covered will now appear wider and shorter. This is a great technique to add fullness to certain areas of the body, such as a small bust.

The inside and outside lines of a garment, such as the seams, bias, and detailing, can give the illusion of a slimmer or curvier figure.

The more uneven the horizontal line is on a garment, the taller and slimmer a garment will look. The more equal it is, the more the area will appear squat or smaller.

Vertical lines which extend from the hem to the torso are more slimming than vertical interrupted lines.

Diagonal lines are slenderizing. Diagonal lines that gather into an arrowhead are more slimming than those which form a V because they draw the viewer's eye upward.

Texture

Texture refers to the surface of the fabric. Fabrics with a lot of texture, such as wool, tweeds, fuzzy mohair and boucle, make that area appear larger. The fabric itself has bulk, and therefore adds bulk to the silhouette.

Smooth fabrics have the opposite effect. They help minimize the covered area. Examples of some of these fabrics are satins, gabardines, matte jerseys and poplins.

Another aspect of texture to consider is whether the fabric is shiny or dull. Shiny fabrics have the same effect as light fabrics because the shine reflects light, making the object appear fuller. Dull fabrics have the same effect as dark fabrics because they absorb light, making the object appear smaller.

The correct combination of color, lines and textures can help you create the look you are aiming for. And combination is key. Do not make the mistake of creating a wardrobe full of dark colors, vertical lines and dull fabrics just so that you can look slim. This will make for a very BORING wardrobe. Balance is the key to creating a beautiful and stylish wardrobe.

"Delete the negative; accentuate the positive!"

– Donna Karan

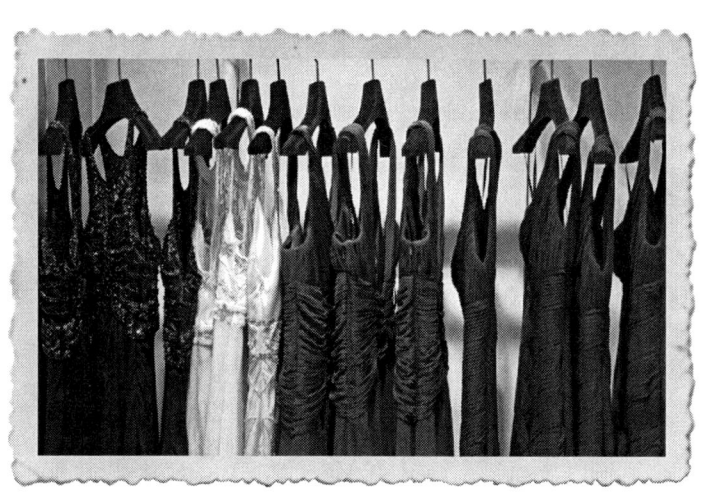

Day 5

"The difference between style and fashion is quality."

– Giorgio Armani

Stylish Closets

I know you don't want to think about it, but in order to move forward you need to take a step back. Yes, you need to step back and take a look at your closet. I am sure you look at your closet many times and think, "I don't have a thing to wear!" Then there are the times when you look frantically for the blouse or perfectly fitting jeans, but can't seem to find it in your overcrowded closet.

The thought of cleaning out your closet is probably sending chills up your spine. I get it. Every time you try to clean it out, you get overwhelmed and just leave it for another day. Well, no more procrastinating. This is the day that you roll up your sleeves and get it done!

OK! LET'S GET STARTED…

You will need to get yourself ready to start trying on your clothes. If that thought makes you cringe…well…that should be a hint of what is in your closet, and that may not be good. I suggest that you put on your best undergarments. Pull your hair back if you have to, in order to keep it off your face and stay cool. You might work up a sweat!

I would not try to tackle your entire wardrobe at once. Instead, do one season at a time. Start with the current season. Take them out of your closet and rearrange your clothes into these categories: jackets, tops, pants, skirts and dresses.

Once that is done, put each category into color stories. For example, all your black pants go together followed by all your gray pants and then jeans and so on, up through the lighter color shades. You will do the same with tops, skirts, dresses and jackets.

I find this is the best way to look at a closet's contents. This organization will give you a better idea of what your buying patterns are. Is your wardrobe filled with black clothes or jeans-and-t-shirts? Is it 80% trousers, but you have great legs that you should be showing off? Whatever your issue, you will be able to see it more clearly by looking at your closet's contents organized in this way.

But do not stop there. You will need to organize your shoes and handbags, too. Follow the same system as your clothes. Separate shoes by pumps, sandals, boots and then by color and heel size. Your handbags need to be filed by color and size as well.

Ok, now it's time to start trying on your clothes. **Look at your wardrobe in a new way, using all the tips that you have learned about dressing for your body type and your coloring.** Make sure you can see yourself in a full-length mirror. Look at yourself objectively but compassionately. This might be an emotional journey for you.

Make sure that the garment fits properly, the color is good for you and that it reflects the image you wish to portray. A good fitting garment should not be too loose and baggy, because this will make you look sloppy and heavier. You also do not want it to fit tightly causing pulls, because this will also make you look heavier.

You will need to put in your closet only the items that fit perfectly well and, of course, look stylish. Keeping your closet organized in categories and color stories will make getting dressed and finding items much easier.

Make two piles of the remaining clothing, one pile for items that you will give away and the other for garments that you need to have altered before you can wear them. *Do not put any items in these piles back in your closet.* The minute you put something back, you will just create the same problem you had before.

To make this process easier, keep in mind the 80/20 rule. You might have heard of it. This is the law of the vital few: 80% of the effects comes from 20% of the causes. Clearly stated when it comes to your wardrobe, you wear 20% of your clothes 80% of the time. What is the 20% I wear 80% of the time? What is the purpose of the rest of my stuff? What can I make room for? Keeping this in mind will make this process easier.

Ok now take a step back and look at your newly organized closet. What do you think?

*"Fashion is architecture:
it is a matter of proportions."*

– Coco Chanel

10 Rules to follow when cleaning your closet.

1. Work *only* on the current season's items.
2. How long has it been since you last wore that item? If longer than 1 year, toss it.
3. How does this garment make you feel when you wear it? If the answer is not great, get rid of it.
4. Does it fit? Not will it fit if you loose 5 pounds. If it does not fit right now, get rid of it. Keeping garments that are the wrong size will simply make you feel bad about who you are not, instead of feeling good about who you are *right now*.
5. Does this garment have any emotional attachment? *Example:* a dress worn on my first date with my ex-husband. Now think about it for a minute: Is it the memory you are holding on to, or the actual garment? If the answer is the memory, take a picture of it and of you wearing it, and, you guessed it: get rid of it.
6. Do I love this item? Do I like it? Or I can take-it-or-leave-it? If you do not love it, yes, get rid of it.
7. Does this color work for me? If the color makes you look sallow or tired and the garment is not that great fitting, toss it. *However,* if the color is not that great but the garment fits beautifully and makes you feel fabulous, consider adding the right colored accessories that might brighten you up.
8. Sort the items that you are keeping in your closet by category and color.
9. Remember to: 1) donate items you no longer need, and 2) take items to be altered to the tailor.
10. Most importantly, have fun trying things on. Play a little!

Let's review:

Put back in your closet **only the items that fit perfectly well and are stylish**. Remember, a good fitting garment should not be too loose and baggy, because this will make you look sloppy and heavier. But you also do not want them to fit too snugly, causing pulls, because this will also make you look heavier.

Make two piles of the remaining clothing: one pile for items that you will give away and the other for those that you need to have altered in order to wear them properly. **Do not put any items in these piles back in your closet.** The minute you put these ill-fitting, unstylish, or oddly-colored clothes back in your closet, you will just create the same problem you had before.

To make the process a little easier, keep in mind **The 80/20 Rule**. You might have heard of it. This is the law of the vital few: in life 80% of the effects comes from 20% of the causes. Clearly stated when it comes to your wardrobe, you wear 20% of your clothes 80% of the time. Keep this in mind when cleaning out your closet. What is the 20% I wear 80% of the time? What is the purpose of the rest of my stuff? What can I make room for?

Ok. Now take a step back and look at your newly organized closet.

What do you think? I am sure it is a hundred times better than before and that you are feeling pretty good right now. Now you need to keep it this way. Remember to keep your closet organized in categories and color stories. That way, getting dressed and finding items will be so much easier.

Closet Clean out List:
What I own after my clean out.

My 20% items are:

My 80% items are:

After looking at my closet I would like to replace the following items:

1. _____
2. _____
3. _____
4. _____
5. _____
6. _____
7. _____

I would love to own the following items:

1. _____
2. _____
3. _____
4. _____
5. _____
6. _____
7. _____

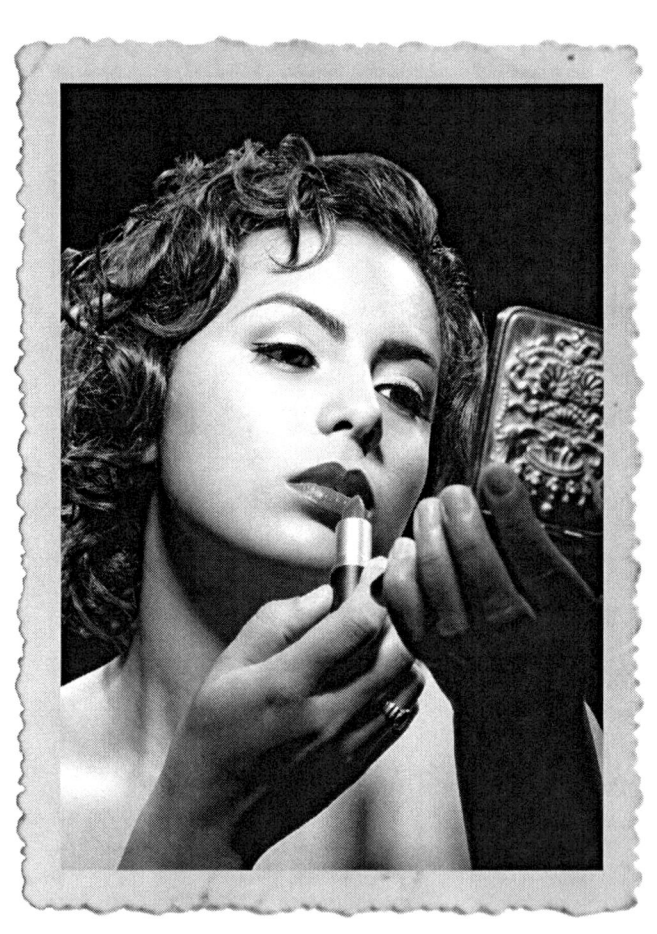

Day 6

*"The best thing is to look natural,
but it takes makeup to look natural."*

– Calvin Klein

Let's Make-Up

In order to get a complete style makeover, you will need to renew your make-up look. I know you are most likely thinking that you are fine in this area of your style, but the reality is, we all need a new look every season. Just like our wardrobes, our cosmetics also need an update.

Does your current make-up live up to your style vision?

Women usually fall into three make-up personalities. The first is the natural woman. She believes that the no make-up look is easy and perfectly acceptable. The second is the woman that can't be seen without a stitch of make-up. She needs to be perfectly polished all the time. The third is where most women fall. It is the woman who loves cosmetics, buys them, but usually won't wear half of what is in her make-up bag.

There really are few women that know how to apply their make-up correctly and know when to replenish it to get a new look. I am not going to attempt to give you a make-up lesson, as that would be a very difficult thing to do without seeing your face. What I will suggest, though, is that you make an appointment with a professional make-up artist who can teach you how to get the look at home.

Before you go, there are a few steps that you can take to get yourself ready for your make-up makeover.

Let's Make-Up A Plan

The first thing you will have to do is clean out your make-up bag.

I know, I know. You thought you were through with cleaning. I promise, no more cleaning after today. But you will want to rid yourself of whatever you do not wear and everything that has been sitting there for more than one year. Bacteria multiply and build up in all make-up and skin care products. Do yourself a favor and throw them out. Keep everything you love that looks great on you. You now know which colors suit you from the Day 4 Color Test.

Once you have cleaned everything out, I want you to make two appointments: one for a facial and the other for a make-up lesson. (If you know how to give yourself a facial, please feel free to do so, but for those of us who love to get pampered, pick up the phone and make the appointment. It is worth it.)

After your skin is clean, you will want to get your make-up done. Make sure that you get a make-up artist that is experienced and has the patience to explain how you can create the look that they have designed for you at home.

Before you head out the door, I suggest that you take a couple of the images of great make-up looks from your Style Vision Board and show them to the make-up artist. This will give the artist a good idea of what you like. The artist will now be able to design a look that reflects your style vision. Once you say OK, the magic will begin! You should be relaxed and artist's attention should be on you.

I love to make this a real experience. My favorite place to go (and I even take my clients there) is the Lancôme boutique in NYC.

I love the products and the service is superb! You will have a wonderful relaxing day with a facial and a make-up application. The best part is that you can actually log on to Lancome-usa.com and watch training videos that give easy-to-follow steps on how to apply the products.

One last note: Nothing says gorgeous more than a beautiful smile. I encourage all of you to try the an at-home teeth whitening products. I will not go into much detail on this aspect, but I encourage you to try the weekly strips and see the difference in seven days. Another alternative is to see your dentist or hygenist. A stylish woman will always have smile for those around her, because she feels good about herself and is able to express it to others.

My Lancôme Favorites

As you know, Lancôme is my skin care and make-up of choice. I just adore the luxurious feel of the products, the research that goes into each one, and the exquisite results. It truly is a line for all ages, skin types, and skin tones. Although it sometimes is a challenge for me to find make-up that matches my skin tone, I always seem to find the perfect shade with Lancôme. Well, let me stop because I truly could go on.

This is my "I can't live without" list. While you might have other skin care and make-up color needs, I wanted to let you into my daily routine in order to give you an idea of why I choose the products and routine that I do. This might help you put together a routine that works for you.

Skin care

Huile Douceur Cleanser- A cleanser and make-up remover in one. You can use just of few drops of Huile Douceur on a damp cotton cloth, and *voila!* Clean face. I love it! My face is fresh with out the tightness that most cleansers cause. My skin feels soft and the fragrance is exquisite.

BiFacil Eye Make-Up Remover- Not only does it remove my eye make-up easily but also my lipstick. It manages to moisturize the area without feeling oily or greasy. So easy to use.

Genefique Eye- The answer to all your eye needs: dark circles and wrinkles seem to disappear. An added bonus is that it is extremely gentle to sensitive skin.

Genefique Concentrate- Lancôme calls it a "youth activator" and it is. The best part is that you will see results in 7 days. I notice my skin looks fresher, and not as dull or tired, when I use it. This is a definite must-have item in my travel bag. Right before boarding, I put some on to hydrate my skin during the flight. I get to my destination looking refreshed.

Absolue Premium BX moisturizer- Yes, this is an anti-aging lotion and I need it. A light weight lotion, it really does moisturize the skin. I love the fact that it has an SPF 15 because that is one less product to apply. The best part is that it leaves your skin looking radiant. I am all about hydration and radiance!

My skin routine in a nutshell: remove all my eye make-up first with BiFacil. Cleanse my face with Huile Douceur. Apply my Genefique eye cream and Genifique Concentrate and end it with Absolue Premium BX moisturizer. Total time spent: 10 minutes! My morning routine is even quicker— half the time— because I will usually just rinse my face with cold water and apply all my moisturizers.

Make-Up

Maquicomplet Concealer- Concealer is a girl's best friend. This concealer is very light weight but covers everything. The best part is its hydrating and anti-oxidant protection.

Oscillation PowderFoundation- I love this mineral powder! Very light weight and comes with a fun-to-use micro-vibrating applicator, it covers everything. The special applicator creates a truly finished look. My skin tends to be dry, but the powder's vitamin E and aloe conditions it, leaving it soft.

Aquatique Eyecolor Base- I actually will wear this smooth eye base alone. It makes my eyes look bright and alive. Use it when applying eyeshadow as well, because it gives a nice clean slate to work with and the color will last longer.

Color Design Eye Shadow- When I want to wear more color, I use these eyeshadow palettes. They are easy to apply and blend, so that you can play with all the great colors. My favorite color is Snap, a taupe/mauve that goes with everything I wear and looks natural.

Le Crayon Khol- Eyeliner is a must for me. What I like about this particular liner is that it stays put. I do not have to worry about it smudging or getting the dreaded raccoon eyes. My favorite color is Black Coffee.

Hypnose Drama Mascara- All I can say is it delivers on its promise. You will get voluminous and thick lashes with just one stroke.

Modele Sourcils Eye Brow Groomer- Creating a natural eyebrow with this tool is easy. It actually combs and colors brows to make them look fresh and polished. My color is Brunet.

La Laque Fever- You have a choice. You can think of this as a lip color with great gloss or a gloss with rich color. I love it because it is easy to use and does double duty: gloss and color. My everyday color is Chromed Pink.

L'Absolu Rouge- I love red lipstick. I think the right red looks great on all women. Red is sexy and seductive. What has stopped me in the past from wearing red is how the color usually bleeds and ends up on my teeth. I am not sure how Lancome does it, but this lipstick stays on for hours, never bleeds or sticks to my teeth. What can I say...I am in love! My color is Absolu Rouge.

Le Crayon Lip Pencil and Lip Liner- I will usually line my lips in color Stand Out when I am wearing Absolu Rouge. But sometimes, I like to wear this liner as an all over color to get a soft red lip.

Blush Subtil Shimmer- I think by now you know that I like quick, double-duty products. This blush in color Mocha Havana is not only a great blush, but it is also a fabulous contour for my face. So simple, it goes with day and night looks.

Body

Nutrix Body Moisturizer- Super hydrating with a wonderful fragrance, this moisturizer leaves my really dry skin feeling smooth and radiant.

My daily make-up routine is easy and takes me 15 minutes tops. First, I put concealer under eyes and over any spots. I then use **Oscillation PowderFoundation,** followed by **Aquatique Eyecolor Base.** I line my upper lid with **Le Crayon Khol** in black coffee and finish my eyes with **Hypnose Drama Mascara** in extreme black. I contour and color my cheeks with **Blush Subtil Shimmer** in Mocha Havana. The finishing touch: **La Laque Fever** in chromed pink. The key: products that do double-duty, such as the **Aquatique Eyecolor Base**, the **Blush Subtil Shimmer**, and **La Laque Fever**.

This is what truly works for me. I can not emphasis enough how important it is to have professional make up artist help you select products and design a daily routine that works for you. Go have fun with color and make-up! It really is one of the pleasures of being a woman.

Hair Today, Gone Tomorrow

So, do you love your hair? Chances are that you answered no. Most of us do not love our hair, whether it is the color, style, condition or a combination of these things. But the reality is that we can all love our hair. All hair needs is a little TLC. Like your skin, your hair needs to be properly cared for and pampered.

There's a very old saying: your hair is your crowning glory. It is one of the few things that you will cry over if it is cut too short, and yet you will be in heaven when it is coifed to perfection. Many times, we hang on to that perfect hairstyle or hair color from long ago, whether it suites us now or not, because we have no idea where to go from here. We get comfortable. We are stuck.

The right haircut is crucial. A good haircut is not only one that compliments your facial shape but also your hair texture and your lifestyle. In order to get the right mix, you need the right hair stylist.

How do you find the right hairstylist? It's just like finding the right boyfriend or partner: you need to look around.

Every reputable hair salon should offer complimentary consultations. These are 5 minute one-on-one meetings with your potential hair stylist. I suggest that you take pictures of both the color and the styles that you like. Discuss your concerns with the stylist. You should be ready to let them know exactly what you expect from your hairstyle.

I like to let my stylist know that I am not good with using a blow dryer and I prefer hair that is wash-and-dry. This is the kind of information that they need to know in order to give you the right cut. A good haircut should be easy to keep and even looks great grown out.

For the best hairstyle, you will need to trust the stylist and be open to change. Getting a haircut is a very emotional experience for a lot of women. Trust that this person is a professional and ask for advice. Let the stylist guide you. I suggest you take a leap of faith and go for a whole new look. It is your turn to shine.

Your Beauty Plan

My current hair and make-up styles are:

The make-up looks I admire the most are:

The ideal make-up routine for me would be:

The hairstyles I admire the most are:

My ideal hairstyle would be:

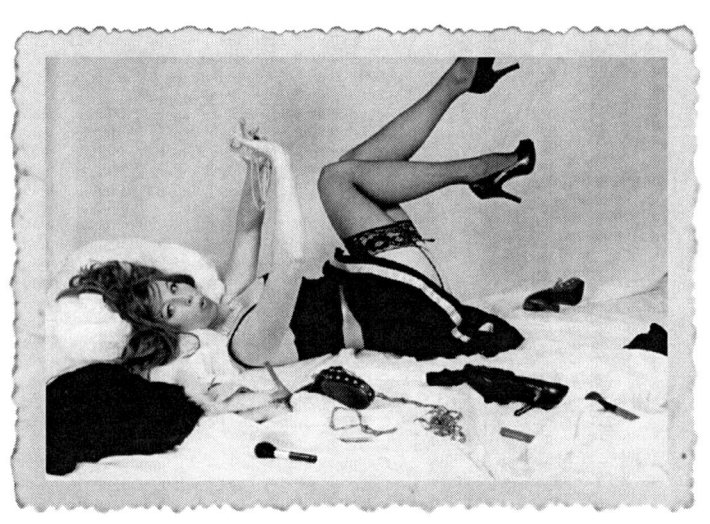

Day 7

*"Please do not have a fit in the fitting room.
Your fashion life begins there."*

Florence Eiseman

Shop Till You Drop

Your previous day started with a makeup lesson and a fantastic look. You got a hair consultation and hopefully were brave enough to get a new hairstyle. So now get your gorgeous self out the door and into a shop!

Shopping should not be stressful. The first thing you need to remember is that size does not matter. Designers size garments differently and you may be an American size 8 and a European size 12. There are times that you may vary in size within the same designer brand. This is because designers often use different factories to produce their garments. So stop obsessing over size and start obsessing about looking good. Do not get discouraged; the worst thing you could do is categorize yourself as a size number.

Do yourself a favor, and put your weight issues aside. I know weight is an issue for all of us at one point or another, but you will need to set these issue aside for today. Remember instead the music that your body is playing and go with it.

If it helps, start your day by going for a workout before you go shopping. I know you might think I am crazy, but trust me. The endorphins you produce during exercise will make you feel good about yourself. Not only that, but you are doing something good for yourself just by going for a walk or taking a great yoga class.

You will also need to prep yourself before going out to shop by wearing the appropriate lingerie. I suggest you go for function this time, and not sexy. I adore sexiness lingerie and wear it whenever I can. I am one of those women who loves to match her bra and panty. But, I am realistic and know that we all need a little help with our curves in order to wear certain styles. This is the reason I am in love with Spanx. They shape your body in a way that is natural and comfortable. I suggest you get a professional bra fitting as well. When you shop wear a skin-tone color bra that fits you perfectly. The smoother your lines are before you start dressing, the easier the experience will be.

Shopping Plan

Great! You are ready to go out there and shop till you drop. WAIT! Don't go out there without a plan. You need to know what you are getting and why. No more ill-fitting clothes, wrong colors and all-around bad choices.

So what make something worth the money and time? My first rule of thumb: **Quality over quantity anytime.** It was the first lesson I learned about style and it is the one I teach my clients. But, there is a time for cheaper pieces and that is when you are purchasing trendy things. These are pieces you can change quickly and only need to last you a season or two. Your quality items, on the other hand, are the ones that are an investment and should be your classic pieces that you will enjoy for a long time. You will save money on these in the long run, because they will last for years.

First let me give you some points on how to tell a quality item:

Fabric is the number one thing to look for. Natural fibers are better quality than man made fibers. Natural fibers include cotton, wool, alpaca, cashmere, linen, silk and bamboo. Man made fibers include polyester, acrylic, nylon and rayon.

Next, look at the **cut and make** of the garment. On a patterned garment, such as plaids and checks, see if the pattern matches at the seams. A well made garment will always match at the seams. For example on a plaid skirt, you should be able to see the plaid match all around. Check for loose threads and any messy sewing, because these are signs of a cheaply made garment. Lastly check the garment's lining. Better garments will have linings that fit like a good slip. Linings should not be tighter or significantly shorter than the garment, and should not have strings attaching them to the garment.

Now you need to determine which garments will be your quality pieces. These should be your anchor pieces, also known as your core wardrobe. They are the items that you will wear 80% of the time. They are the pieces you will build your wardrobe around. You will need these to be classic pieces, not trend pieces. Since they are classic pieces, they are also the items you want to spend most of your money on.

The following is a great formula to use when deciding how much to spend on an item:

Take the cost of the item and divide by the number of times you think you will wear it.

Let's use as an example a pair of black light weight wool trousers. Suppose you find a pair of classic trousers at $240. You will most likely wear these pants twice a week for about 50 weeks of the year so that is roughly 100 times.

$240 divided by 100 = $2.40 per wear/per year.

Since this is a quality garment you should have it for minimum of three years.

$2.40 divided by 3 = $0.80. That is less than a dollar per wear.

I think that is totally worth it!

Now if you are thinking of purchasing a very trendy item that you will wear for only a season or two, do not spend the money. The likelihood of that garment looking dated quickly is high. Unless you can extend its life by wearing it with different items to make it look updated, don't bother. Save your money.

List of anchor pieces that every wardrobe should have.

Remember these are the pieces that you need to invest in. Every woman should have the following garments in your closet. The style details will depend on her shape and personal style.

1. **The LBD:** Yes, the "little black dress" made famous by one of my favorite designers, Coco Chanel. This is the short cocktail dress in a good fabric that can take you from day to night.

2. **White Shirt:** A crisp white shirt make of quality cotton. The shirt should fit you perfectly and could be worn tucked in or worn out.

3. **Black Trousers:** Trousers should be of a light weight wool that can be worn 9 months of the year. If you live in a warm climate, they can be of made of cotton/lycra blend to keep you cool. The best style to get is a straight leg classic fit.

4. **Black Skirt:** Make sure that it is made from a year round fabric. Here you can choose between the A-line style or pencil skirt. I love pencil skirts because I think they are a sexy feminine line.

5. **The Sexy Dress**: The dress you wear to go on a date or just to feel super sexy. Try choosing the shade of red that works best for your skin tone. Red is associated with love and passion. If you feel intimidated by red, use another color within your color palette. The point is to memorable in a classy way.

6. **Blazer**: A nice fitting classic blazer that can be part of a suit with either trousers or a skirt. I like a nice feminine line for this garment. The details should all be impeccably made.

7. **Coat**: If you live in a cold climate, your coat is the first garment others see when you are busy walking around. You want a great fitting wool coat. Here again, a nice

feminine line will make you look more elegant and pulled-together than a straight shapeless style. Pick either a neutral color or a flash of color that works with your wardrobe. Try a red, blue, green or purple coat, depending on your coloring.

8. **Trench coat**: This is your warm weather and rain coat. There are so many options for different trench coat styles today. You have many to choose from, but keep in mind your "melody". Some cuts will look better than others. Follow the same rules of color as your winter coat.

9. **Jeans**: Nothing looks better than a great fitting pair of jeans. Try a classic boot cut in a dark denim. This jeans style looks great on everyone and will last past the current trend. Dark denim can be dressed down or dressed up. You might even be able to wear them to work, depending on your office dress policy.

10. **Sweater**: A cashmere sweater should be part of every woman's wardrobe. I love the slightly oversized cardigan. I love the casual elegant look of a sweater that can be worn as jacket. You can also make it a V-neck, turtleneck, mock turtle, crew neck–whatever feels right to you. Start by buying one, and then add them gradually to your wardrobe.

11. **T-shirt**: A good quality t-shirt made of a great cotton/lycra fabric that can be layered or worn alone. Keep the color neutral so that you can wear it with all the items in your wardrobe.

12. **Lingerie**: A basic staple to your wardrobe should be the great fitting skin-tone colored bra and panty. These undergarments should support you and give you a smooth line underneath your clothes. You can then build your lingerie wardrobe to include sexy pieces that fit and flatter you.

13. **Shoes & Handbags**: Finally, what we all love: shoes

and handbags! Here again go for quality over quantity. Get a great pair of neutral colored shoes and handbag. You will be able to wear them with everything in your wardrobe and they will be worth every cent.

14. **Eyewear:** Both eyeglass and sunglasses are an important part of your look. Jackie-O made it her signature, and so can you. Make sure that you get a pair that flatters your face's shape and skin coloring. Your personality plays an important part of your eyewear choice as well. Bolder personalities can get away with bolder frames.

Stylish shopping list.

Now you know the items you have in your closet and your must-haves. You are ready to make a list of that one ideal outfit you are going to shop for!

List the items you have:

ITEM	COLOR	STYLE	OCCASION
EX: PANTS	BLACK	TROUSERS	WORK

List items you need to buy:

ITEM	COLOR	STYLE	OCCASION	PRICE

Now you know the style lines, textures and colors that you should be looking for. You know the items that you need to shop for and why. When you go shopping, you will need to take your Style Vision Board picture and your Style Statement. You will be able to refer to them when you need to, and they will keep you focused. Put on your great fitting lingerie, preferably in a skin-tone color and with good support. Wear comfortable shoes to walk around in, but make sure to carry a pair of nice heels to wear when trying on clothes. (The better boutiques and department stores usually will have a pair of heels for you to try on.)

At this point I want to mention a little bit about the shopping experience. When I was in my twenties, I used to go to a neighborhood boutique with my mom and sister. They gave us such fantastic customer service that I always came out looking great and buying something. The experience was everything I wanted and enjoyed. Each and every time, these ladies made always made me feel comfortable and suggested we play a little with looks and styles. I still have a few outfits I bought there. They are classic pieces that look fantastic to this day.

I love the old world charm of being catered to when shopping: the private dressing rooms with a sales person that focuses only on your needs. The glass of water or coffee ready for you so that you are hydrated and comfortable. The occasional glass of wine or champagne doesn't hurt either.

I love to give my clients this experience. I make sure that not only the product but also the customer service is excellent. Everywhere I take them treats them wonderfully. We all should have this treatment when shopping. Make sure you find places that treat you like a million dollars, even if you only spend a hundred.

Shop just for one great outfit today. This outfit should be a reflection of your new style. Do not overwhelm yourself with trying to tackle a whole new wardrobe. Remember, this is your *7 Days to Style*, so the goal is to be stylish, and not to have a closet full of clothes. You are looking for the one outfit that expresses your essence.

Ask for help from a salesperson you feel comfortable with and whose style you like. Let that person know that you would like a new look, and that you are shopping for one outfit only, and not an entire wardrobe. You do not want a salesperson that is only looking to make multiple sales. You want someone who truly cares. Pull out an example from your Style Vision Board. Have fun and play with different looks.

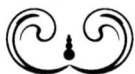

*"Luxury must be comfortable,
otherwise it is not luxury."*

– Coco Chanel

Designers I Love

You already know that I have always been a dreamer. As a teenager, my dream and vision for myself was as a fashion designer. I saw myself creating the most beautiful outfits and living a very glamorous life. Coco Chanel was my icon. She was the reason I started wearing menswear accessorized with pearls and bows as a teen. (I know it sounds very chic when you picture Coco doing that, but trust me. It was not so chic when I did it.)

I knew I was off to a good start, career wise – I was one of the best in my high school fashion sketching class, as a matter of fact. The next step was learning to sew. I was psyched! I took a sewing class at our local Singer store, but I was shocked at how difficult it was! My mom and grandmother made it look so easy. Why was I not getting it!?! My mom gave it to me straight, one more time. "Monica, you're not good at sewing. You need to practice sewing everyday, or you won't make a good designer."

My dream was shattered. There went my glamorous career. I was disappointed because honestly, the thought of sewing everyday did not make me happy.

I did not become a fashion designer. My life is not as glamorous as I pictured it to be as a teenager, living on the French Riviera sipping vintage Veuve Cliquot, but it is pretty damned good. I became a textile designer, and I founded my own personal styling consultancy in NYC. And yes, I do drink Veuve Cliquot and I have been to the French Riviera.

I tell you this story because I have a deep respect and appreciation for fashion designers' talent and hard work. Their ability to envision a beautiful design, construct each and every part, and then assemble the components to create a perfectly finished piece amazes me. It is truly an art.

There are so many designers I love I found it extremely difficult to sit down and pick my top ones to feature in this book. I am still in love with the house of Coco Chanel. Her vision of women and fashion are still relevant today. You may have noticed that I use more than one of her quotes; she was a true visionary.

As for contemporary designers, here are some of my favorites:

Catherine Malandrino designs sexy functional clothing. Known for beautiful knitwear, she makes some of the most well crafted knit pieces. I own a few of her pieces and love to take clients to her boutique because I know I can find that sexy date dress there and a lot more. As a matter of fact, the dress I am wearing in the Ch. 1 photo is a Catherine Malandrino!

Marc Jacobs starts trends and fashion movements, such grunge chic. His clothing is fun and makes people see the art in fashion. I love all three collections he designs: Marc Jacobs collection, the Marc line, and Louis Vuitton.

Oscar de la Renta - Romance and elegance are always key in his collections. If you want to look like a member of the real "ladies who lunch", Oscar is the true *caballero* (gentleman) that knows how to dress them. He dressed Jackie O, the American queen of fashion.

Roland Mouret - This Frenchman dresses women in a sexy and sophisticated fashion. He is known for his sexy form fitting dresses designed to fit like a glove. Even when he drapes a garment, it looks sexy.

Christopher Bailey - The designer for *Burberry Prorsum* that has taken this traditional, classic label to a young and very hip collection. He has a definite gift for design. I love how he plays with fabric textures and shapes to make collections look fresh.

Alber Elbaz - Designing for the house of *Lanvin,* he creates beautiful collections that are always clean and feminine with very interesting shapes.

Ralph Lauren - He is always true to himself and his customer. I think there is never mistaking a Ralph Lauren collection. You can always trust Ralph Lauren will deliver true American sportswear.

I will stop at lucky number seven.

"Clothes are my passion and my knowledge. I've studied fashion from every angle- historically and critically, cerebrally and emotionally. "

– Vera Wang

You Look Marvelous!

So this is the end of your *7 Days to Style*. You have worked so hard and learned so much about yourself. Hopefully you have followed the book and done all the exercises. If you haven't, what are you waiting for!?!

I have given you all the tools you need to start being that fabulously stylish lady you are meant to be. I am sure that you look marvelous and feel fantastic. You should have cleaned out all the old baggage – physical and emotional – that was keeping you from your authenticity and discovered your true self.

Remember, being stylish is not necessarily being "in fashion" or wearing the most expensive clothing. You should know by now that being stylish is about knowing who you are, loving who you are and knowing how to communicate this with your clothing choices. The person that screams for attention either verbally or non-verbally via body language or choice of clothing is someone that does not exude style. The same goes for the person that tries to hide, blend in and go unnoticed. The woman who owns her space, walks with confidence and wears clothing that exudes elegance is a Stylish woman.

If you feel that you might need to reread the book and do the exercises again, that is ok. We all have different ways of learning and different ways of absorbing information. Still, you owe it to yourself to consider how you feel about yourself today and how you want to feel about yourself for the rest of your life.

The subtitle of this book is "A Guide to Your Authentic Style". Authenticity, or your uniqueness, is what sets us apart from each other. It is that essence that I try to extract from each of you so that you can exude YOUR style.

I invite you to have fun in this journey and maybe take a friend or two along with you. Discovering your style and helping a friend discover hers is more exciting than going at it along. Aren't all journeys more fun with a companion? This is the purpose of my Style Workshops: to share the experience and have fun.

I would love to hear your comments regarding the book and your new style. You can email me at Monica@stylemattersonline.com

I wish that you all have that confidence to look at yourselves in the mirror and say, "This is who I am. I love the music my body plays, I am worth the best, I love how I look and I LOVE ME!"

My glass is raised to all the stylish women this book has helped to create.

May you always enjoy the music your body plays and live your life with Style!

XOXO,
Monica

7 Days To Style To Do's

Day 1
-
-
-

Day 2
-
-
-

Day 3
-
-
-

Day 4
-
-
-

Day 5
-
-
-

Day 6
-
-
-

Day 7
-
-
-

Style Notes

About Monica

Monica Diaz, personal stylist and founder of New York-based personal image consultancy **Style Matters, Inc.**, has worked in nearly every sector of the fashion industry from product development to merchandising, sales, and buying for more than 20 years.

Initially specializing in textile designs, Monica's creations were well sought after by Ralph Lauren, Oscar de la Renta, Carolina Herrera, J. Crew, Banana Republic, Jones New York, Hart, Schaffner & Marx and others.

Recruited by Bergdorf Goodman, Monica directed merchandising and purchasing decisions for seasonal collections for the Marc Jacobs boutique. At Oxford Industries, a leading menswear manufacturer for both private and brand name labels, Monica specialized in product design and development.

Featured in Glow magazine as one of the Best of Manhattan for her personal styling services, Monica also appeared on Univision's morning show *Al Despertar* as a fashion and style expert advising about appropriate office wear.

Monica holds degrees in both Textile Technology and Fashion Marketing from Fashion Institute of Technology, New York City.

Style Matters, Inc. offers private consultations, corporate seminars and personalized workshops, helping men and women discern their personal styles, express their inner goals, and create their own distinct fashion image.

www.stylemattersonline.com